LANGPORT

Please return/renew this item by the last date shown on this label, or on your self-service receipt.

To renew this item, visit **www.librarieswest.org.uk** or contact your library

Your borrower number and PIN are required.

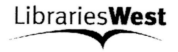

Libraries**West**

1

4 6 0324765 7

Edward D. Nelson

Table of Contents

Attention Deficit Hyperactivity

: An Introduction

How Does Attention Deficit Disorder Affect Daily Life?

Therapies for ADHD: Medications

How Is ADD Distinct From ADHD?

The Many Ways That ADD May Present In Children

Getting Your Information Correct About Attention Deficit Disorder.

Is it really attention deficit disorder?

What Is Attention Deficit Hyperactivity Disorder?

Six suggestions for calming the ADD brain

What Is Attention Deficit Disorder, Anyway?

How Does ADD Impact Your Child's Education And Schooling?

The Gift Of Resilience And ADD

How To Effectively Arrange Your Child's Therapy For ADHD

How Does Attention Deficit Disorder Affect Daily Life?

Hyperactive Attention Deficit Disorder the substitute

How Is Attention Deficit Disorder (ADD) Diagnosed?

What Does An Attention Deficit Disorder Diagnose Really Mean?

ADHD Treatment: Getting Started

Medications for ADHD: A Summary

Therapies for ADHD: Medications

What Takes Place Throughout ADHD Treatments When

Medication Is Insufficient?
Therapies for ADHD: The Diet
The Negative Effects Of ADHD Therapies

Attention Deficit Hyperactivity: An Introduction

ADHD has many structures and various marginally contrasting appearances. There are now more than five recorded and reported types of ADHD.

Furthermore, albeit here and there addressed, it is broadly recognized that this is an ailment which is helped through the qualities, and subsequently frequently shows itself as specific problems of the sensory system (of which there are a large number).

The DSM-IV Manual of Determination reports that any sort, structure or sort of Consideration Shortage Hyperactivity Turmoil ought to be gathered under the class of ADHD. This really focal rundown is in this manner broken into ADHD types;

- ADHD Joined Type
- Hasty Hyperactive Sort or
- ADHD Heedless Sort

Some time prior, the expressions a lack of ability to concentrate consistently jumble "with" or "without" hyperactivity were moreover instituted and broadly utilized. There can be numerous blends so various victims will show various side effects.

For the most part Consideration Deficiency
Hyperactivity influences various areas of the cerebrum,
frequently more than
four remarkable pieces of the cerebrum. Along these
lines, it brings about numerous special "profiles" and
"styles" of
youngsters, so having a 'standard arrangement of
conduct and observing against that for any kid
furthermore, potentially even grown-ups with ADHD or
ADD doesn't necessarily in every case work.
There are four primary circles:

1) Failure to join in
2) Challenges with Motivation Control
3) Issues related with engine fretfulness and additionally
hyperactivity
4) An expanded penchant to become exhausted - A
condition yet to be "formally" pronounced in
manuals of finding

The following are a couple of additional significant
components of this condition:

a. At the point when you know what to search for, this
issue and its belongings are detectable and can be
observed by and large, yet this ought to be done both at
school and at home. If a youngster
shows side effects just in one spot then perhaps there is
a justification for this which ought to be

researched.

b. frequently, the problem turns out to be more recognizable before the youngster arrives at seven years old.
Since ADHD is created to some extent by neurological issues, it could be from a head injury or
may have been conveyed in the hereditary qualities itself.
In the event that ADHD will happen typically it will be evident by the age of seven.

How Does Attention Deficit Disorder Affect Daily Life?

Living with ADD may not be simple for any youngster, teen or grown-up who has been determined to have ADD. An individual as of late determined to have ADD and foreseeing the remainder of their life may not be simple
for them. They might be uncertain the way that their illness will be impacted by age. However, over the long haul
what's more, you mature with your insight, you begin to comprehend ways of taking care of the side effects of furthermore, successfully manage ADD.

Youngsters with ADD can be neglectful, uninformed about the impacts of their activities on others and crazy, or they may effectively get diverted. They could show an excessive number of their sentiments or movement to other people. Furthermore, the side effects will remain very reliable in any event, when they go through
different ages. Anyway their capacity to deal with these side effects will work on after some time, as they get more established.

The manner in which ADD can affect on your life will to a great not set in stone by what medicine you select to treat the issue. You could wish to counsel a specialist to give yourself a superior comprehension representing things to come impacts that taking energizers could have, and furthermore different ramifications of taking meds.

There are numerous qualities and characteristics which are average of ADD. Individuals experiencing it ought to be ready for these. These may be troubles in their being excessively mindful of subtleties, or on the other hand issue with keeping quiet and for any time span. They may be nervous or have issues having the option to push on through and complete any given errand.

By the by it is feasible to do a scope of things to relieve the way of behaving so frequently connected with ADD. It is feasible to turn out to be more coordinated and more controlled in holding things under control. You can pick any book or a schedule to help you, however the cycle is significant.

Schedules, timetables and arranging ought to be utilized broadly as these will show you control. As a victim of ADD you will be normally disposed to neglect, let completely go and be reckless. By utilizing a straightforward gadget, for example, a schedule you will act in a more controlled way, in a way dissimilar to your real essence. Hence you will commit less errors. You could likewise wish to turn into a piece of a gathering as this will offer Extra help. You might feel the requirement for somebody to trust in, who can comprehend you circumstance well. An individual with ADD could be an ideal sidekick since they might have the option to interface with you better than any companion or a relative, since they can uphold you just as far as possible.

Therapies for ADHD: Medications

ADHD medicines frequently incorporate some type of treatment drug. There are a few
prescriptions available that are utilized broadly to assist youngsters as well as grown-ups who with having
been determined to have treatment. A considerable lot of these treatment choices are dependent upon the person's
response to them. In some cases this implies that you should attempt a few preceding seeing as the right
decision for your condition. Finding the right medicine implies that ADHD can be to a lesser degree a
issue for the individual and they can work on their everyday capabilities, particularly at school
or on the other hand work.

Most drugs for ADHD are energizers. Numerous people don't grasp this as numerous
that experience the ill effects of ADHD are very twisted up and worked up. However, dissimilar to those that would take a
energizer to give them more energy, the energizers work another way for the individual with
ADHD. They work by invigorating the mind in a particular region to assist them with acquiring advantages such

as better abilities to focus, more control rather than drive choices and more clarity of mind in the undertakings
they need to achieve. These prescriptions work by assisting the cerebrum with having more prominent self guideline.

Here are the absolute most normal meds for ADHD medicines.
Methylphenidate: These are tracked down in Ritalin, Metadate, Methylin and Focalin. These are
typically required three times each day after feasts. There are others including Ritalin LA and Focalin
XR that are long portions that will reach out as long as 12 hours.

Amphetamines: Here, you might find decisions, for example, Dexedrine that is taken a few times for every day, ADDerall which is both accessible in short and longer periods and others.
Different drugs for ADHD treatment including Atomoxetine, Bupropion which is all the more well known as Wellbutrin, Benzphetamine which is significantly less strong, Provigil which is a new decision, and Clonidine.

There is a ton of experimentation that goes into the assurance of the right drug for an
person that experiences ADHD. The best instrument that can be given to them is exact

analysis as well as determination at taking the prescriptions. When something isn't right with the prescription, they ought to tell their PCP at that moment so an option can be
found. ADHD medicines with prescription ought to likewise be assisted with conduct and instructive help too. The blend can permit youngsters and grown-ups to track down additional responses to their questions and generally speaking improved results to their requirements.

How Is ADD Distinct From ADHD?

A lack of ability to concentrate consistently Turmoil or ADD is an extremely muddled, and over and over confounded,
jumble. Its start is physiological, yet it can have a large number of results that come
close by with it. That separated, what is the separation among ADHD and ADD? ADHD is the
shortened type of Consideration Shortfall Hyperactive Turmoil, its significant signs being perceptible
hyperactivity and impulsivity. These are the signs that are perceptible to the intentional
spectator. ADD represents A lack of ability to concentrate consistently Turmoil with the significant signs being absence of
focus. Presently a ton of different things can come close by with both of these subtypes of
ADHD, however those are the particular attributes of both.

For a long time, the standard image of A lack of ability to concentrate consistently Turmoil has been the young man that is
skipping off the walls and making his educators and guardians go distraught. ADHD is for certain
the more recognizable of the two subtypes since it is quite a lot more observable than ADD. Since

hyperactivity causes much more disturbance and issues for homerooms, it gets the most notification furthermore, will be gotten on a ton speedier. Unfortunately, regardless of whether ADD is less noticeable, the outcomes
of the problem can similarly as negative.

With careless a lack of ability to concentrate consistently confusion, or ADD, the individual getting through it will give the impression
of being spacey and disarranged. More regularly, casualties with this sort will look out of the
window during classes and won't appear as though they are ever to some degree there. It is considerably more precarious
to make a finding and a many individuals with this type of ADD go a long time without knowing
they have it. Yet, the outcomes of the floating psyche can similarly as belittle.
For quite a while, it was viewed as that just young men experienced ADHD. Nonetheless, this invention
has been busted of late. It is presently recognized that the two young ladies and young men can experience the ill effects of
a lack of ability to concentrate consistently jumble, and many don't receive in return in middle age. One dissimilarity that has
been seen is that young ladies are leaned to have the oblivious rendition of ADD, and ordinarily it
is wrongly analyzed as sorrow. Since oblivious ADD doesn't make recognizable difficulties

furthermore, disturbances to the close by environmental factors, a great deal of them persevere peacefully for quite a long time before they
find the genuine explanation of their situation.

With both ADHD and ADD, making a conclusion from the get-go is exceptionally fundamental. Despite the fact that inconveniences
with schools are the most obvious signs, a few casualties don't dislike getting the everyday schedule. Monitor your kids, scholastically, however by and large
also, mentally too. Do they disapprove of different youngsters? Does maybe they
experience issues taking care of or are very cluttered? Do they experience issues sitting
still for a while? Might it be said that they are incredibly quiet or very loquacious? Presently any of these
signs don't specifically signify ADD or ADHD, yet they truly do highlight requesting outside
help from a specialist or an instructor.

Your youngster's mental prosperity is similarly as in school. Affirm it out assuming you sense like something is off. On the off chance that left for a really long time not analyzed, ADD
can make a great deal of other coming about inconveniences that can consume a large chunk of the day to get freed off and can be
captured.

The Many Ways That ADD May Present In Children

A lack of ability to concentrate consistently Confusion can take a few structures in kids. Following the child is easy
with an extremely turbulent. ADD. Young men for the most part come into this classification. However at that point there are some
sorts of ADD which go undiscovered on the grounds that their belongings in kids are less obviously
obvious. This happens basically if there should arise an occurrence of young ladies.

There are numerous young ladies who are designated "spitfires". They much of the time show a portion of the significant
highlights off ADD, such as being more engaged with proactive tasks, yet not generally so wild as the young men
themselves. Thus educators and guardians rush to make the judgment call that the kid has no
interest in scholastics and is fundamentally not coordinated, however the chance of ADD is only from time to time
thought of.

Other than the "spitfire" types, the "effusive" young ladies could likewise be experiencing ADD, yet at the same excess

undiscovered. This is a combination of over-movement and obliviousness, and is generally promoted as socially outgoing individual. These young ladies are incredibly loquacious than being actually dynamic and can't
quit talking regardless of whether they are totally cautioned. They likewise can't recount stories exhaustively and
will wander from their viewpoints in light of ADD.

Those whom we call as "daydreamers" could likewise be experiencing ADD. They don't draw any consideration regarding themselves and are exceptionally very in nature. In any case, their a lot being into
themselves and not focusing on the class is one more type of ADD, in spite of the
"effusive" young ladies. They might show tension and despondency when given school projects, yet can't finish the ventures due to their absence of fortitude. This by and large goes undiscovered
since the youngster is believed to be lethargic and, guardians and educators neglect to recognize the problem in
time.

Is intriguing that numerous young ladies with ADD have a seriously high pace of intelligence level and could be called

"gifted". At the point when a youngster has a high level of intelligence everything looks great in everyday schedule, their need
escape clauses get reflected as they mature into grown-ups. Remember that ADD isn't a learning confusion, and patients don't unavoidably are unfortunate entertainers in school. Till secondary school they can
be very wealthy, however with mounting tension and tasks side effects might turn out to be more furthermore, more clear. When undiscovered, A lack of ability to concentrate consistently Turmoil might really hurt a person. Kids

will be called disorderly, lacking knowledge and apathetic, when in truth, they may be quiet
victims of ADD. They will have exceptionally low regard of themselves, and trust themselves to be
weaklings or dumb in light of their concerns. It is pivotal that the issue is recognizes and treated
before it turns out to be past the point of no return and any drawn out harm is finished.

Getting Your Information Correct About Attention Deficit Disorder.

With all that is expounded on ADHD, the vast majority of us will generally consider a terrible little chap running about
demolishing whatever comes his direction. So we frequently accept that we can detect the youngster with ADD while
we are out. Well the devious young man is there fine, yet did we at any point spare an idea about the
young lady who sits tranquil and removed with her mom, one who is plainly affable, horribly hesitant to stand up and stalls out mentally when addressed? In all probabilities, everybody would neglect to figure that she may be experiencing ADD or the A lack of ability to concentrate consistently Confusion.

Troublesome as they are, ADD and ADHD have a few clear side effects as well. The impacted individual experiences interruption, simple distraction and low confidence, deals with issue in following quick discussions and gets exceptionally confused with undertakings. ADD and ADHD both can impede mental development in this that the impacted youngster needs to battle with the everyday schedule task cutoff times,

neglecting to complete things on time. These issues likewise loot the youngster off his/her capacity to make due
the possessions and to monitor time.

ADD Side effects:

• Needs force, experiences sloth
• Values others more, regarding their singular cutoff points
• Frequently unassertive or under-emphatic
• An excessive amount of acquiescence
• Unreasonable humbleness and unobtrusiveness
• Clearly affable and bashful
• Keeping away from swarm, liking to remain alone and socially removed
• Not ready to open up effectively and become friends with, in spite of the fact that they make a couple of bonds
Since it is accepted that young ladies are for the most part modest, individuals frequently disregard the ADD side effects in
them and they are left untreated. Their outward quiet, calm and good manners are generally to cover
up the inward unsettling influence. ADD impacted young ladies are close to home and exceptionally delicate to analysis; yet
the sentiments summoned consequently, in the wake of being reprimanded, stay untold. They simply continue with life,

battling quietly. Curiously, their ADHD partners push ahead with totally
no indication of stress or weakness and appear to be absolutely unaffected by all hindrances in the social status. Young ladies experiencing ADD can't endure pressure and ordinarily step back more into a shell with a
conviction that they are worthless and can do nothing right.

Assisting an individual with ADD

All ADD impacted young ladies are dominatingly close to home, independent of their temperament — be it bashful,
social, thoughtful person, hyperactive or super-rash. This over-awareness clearly welcomes normal disturbs which, thus, bring about increasingly more pressure. Thus, they ought to be educated to
oversee pressure through different strategies since the beginning. They should likewise be credited a
certain recovery time to refocus or gather themselves after each harm or profound bombshell.
Despite the fact that it is actually the case that guardians generally hope everything works out for their youngsters, they once in a while,
unwittingly, block mental development in their children by flinging an excessive amount of analysis at them or by making them distraught with a progression of endless do's and don'ts like "You should not be so senseless.

You got to complete school with high grades", "You want to work on your looks. Attempt and be as
shrewd as your sibling", "You ought to be somewhat more self-assured. This won't help", "for what reason do you let
yourself be underestimated? Awaken", "Make more companions", "Don't give up off things so
without any problem" et cetera. While every one of these are fine now and again, a lot of analysis breeds low confidence in her — be she bashful, candid, stepped back or wild!

At school, over the course of the day, the certainty and self-respect of these young ladies are continually
broken and their main relief is at home, where they can revamp their squashed nobility and
revive themselves to battle one more day. Persistent analysis establishes in them the conviction that they
are useless. These young ladies experiencing ADD become incredibly hasty, disarranged and
need center in everything just to get horrible scores in class. Brimming with interruptions, these young ladies need
the force and energy to foster their character and ranges of abilities that their friends have. Rather than
pointing at their constraints, it is smarter to commend them or appreciate when they get a
expertise or give indications of a decent capacity. Their mind simply needs a positive lift. Also, it's not hard
to encourage them — an ADD-impacted young lady can undoubtedly luck out and track down interest in some

movement. That then, at that point, turns into the main positive move, the most wanted defining moment in their lives!

Is it really attention deficit disorder?

Attention Deficit Disorder or ADD is most frequently identified in boys of primary school age.
Indications consist of lack of concentration, being restless, reckless mannerisms, or lack of
focus. But what brings about these indications, in fact? And should every one of the
occurrences of ADD be treated?

In a few occurrences, the indications of ADD may in fact be indicative of a more severe
psychological predicament, such as depression, bipolar disorder, brain defects and even
nervousness. On the other hand, at times the occurrence of the particular inattentive behavior
may simply be due to allergic reactions, sensitivities to the environment, nutritional deficits or
also too much caffeine.

Many times, young boys are wrongly diagnosed with Attention Deficit Disorder merely for
conducting themselves the way anybody would be expecting. Young boys will by and large
make reckless resolutions, have a lot of superfluous energy, cannot sit still, and have short
concentration period in school. Combined with the fact that the majority of school age children

use up more than forty hours a week watching TV and playing computer games, it is not a
surprise that a lot of children have energy to use up.

ADD mannerism is frequently indicative of creativeness, giftedness, high aptitude, and a child
being a visual theorist.

In short, an analysis of Attention Deficit Disorder ought to be thought of as a start, and not an
end. Too frequently, when a doctor sees that a child is agitated and has a short concentration
period, she writes a medication for Dexedrine or Ritalin and that is that. But these drugs have
possibly unsafe side effects, and are not essentially going to cure the predicament at all.

A further comprehensive examination of the occurrence generally falls upon the child's parents.
The facts stated here is aimed to steer the parents in the right track, giving propositions of
where to begin looking for the reason of the child's Attention Deficit Disorder related manners.

What Is Attention Deficit Hyperactivity Disorder?

Consideration Shortfall Hyperactivity Problem or ADHD is a psychological problem, which roughly three to seven percent youngsters are having. Because of this issue youngsters manifest the quality of consistent way of behaving, heaps of action along with frequently being viewed as rebellious. Really that doesn't imply that the individual is terrible however truth be told, they don't have command over their psychological range. They go through absence of focus in light of the fact that at a time they are probably going to think about numerous components rather than one specific component.

This problem is likewise found in numerous grown-ups other than kids. In grown-ups, it is called Grown-up Consideration Shortage Turmoil or AADD. Among all kids determined to have ADHD around 30 to 70 percent will continue with their issue through adulthood. Grown-ups figure out how to live with it and work around it and need less assistance. They can deal with the problem of their own as it's harder to recognize too. However, by and large the two kids and grown-up may require drugs for improved results.

In youngsters this problem gives indications like heedlessness, imprudent way of behaving and a consistent
anxiety. In grown-ups, it is more earnestly to determine yet youngsters to have this problem can't stand by for long. They can't focus on something specific for an extensive stretch of time. In grown-ups, it
becomes troublesome now and again to structure their lives and to design everyday exercises. They don't feel the significance to remain mindful or to quit being anxious on the grounds that these are not by any stretch of the imagination significant
issues for them.

ADHD is a problem for which help of clinical faculty is vital. It tends to be dealt with
be that as it may, can't be relieved completely. For this problem prescription is additionally fundamental.

Six suggestions for calming the ADD brain

On the off chance that you are a grown-up enduring with ADD, you could perceive that in spite of the fact that it is not difficult to say,
dialing back can be a truly challenging in the event that certainly feasible thing to do from the get go.
Regardless of who you are there are various things that must be finished and quite frequently little
time accessible to finish them. So then your psyche begins to work at high velocity trying to
accomplish however much it can and the sky is the limit from there. The outcome can be pressure at not having the option to meet your
prerequisites, prompting you blowing up about the way that it looks unthinkable. Due to
this you go through bunches of time stressing, and sadly brief period having fun.
While dialing back can be something complicated to accomplish it tends to be finished. The following are six laid out
strategies to help you to slow your mind ADD etc.:

1. Put down your work

Set business hours and regardless of what is left by the day's end, leave. Stand by your

rules. Despite the fact that it will appear to be important to stay at work past 40 hours, keep away from it at all expense. You will
work better and all the more proficiently during the more limited hours of the day realizing that you should leave
at a set time. Furthermore, require ends of the week (or if nothing else two or three days seven days off).

2. Focus on a customary commitment

Focus on motivation to escape your home or out of your office every week. You might need to
go to a class, perhaps something that you have for a long time needed to do. Ensure that you 'pay'
ahead of time for the class with the goal that you have motivation to join in.

3. Set up for a break with others

Hardly any things are pretty much as charming as having a night out with companions. This might accompany associates,
with companions, with family, or with individuals from another gathering.

4. Keep a journal

Writing in a journal expects that you stop, ponder what you need to say, and afterward follow up on what you think. It assists you with managing apprehensive strain and accomplish clearness. make a goal to compose consistently - regardless of whether just for a couple of moments!

5. Switch your PC off two hours before bed

Since PCs are a passage to intriguing things, for ADDers you can get yourself
sitting at a PC until the early hours of the morning totally unmindful of what is
occurring around you. To ensure that this doesn't occur to you switch the PC off at
least 2 hours before you intend to nod off in order to reasonably unwind and dial back around evening time.

6. Ponder

There are assorted strategies for reflection, so find one that suits you, yet you might need to
think about care reflection. This is the activity of keeping your brain in the present -
whether you are strolling, working or washing dishes. Try to keep your psyche in the
at this very moment not the past or future.

It is fine to begin doing this gradually, with short meetings spent in careful contemplation day to day (perhaps just 5 minutes all at once), after that building your exhibition as you become more quiet.

What Is Attention Deficit Disorder, Anyway?

As parents, I am sure that many of you will have spent sleepless nights concerned that the
strange behavior our child exhibited today may be the first signs of Attention Deficit Disorder.
Our concerns are justified in many ways as most of us believe we know the fundamental signs
of the disease are, and we obviously panic at the thought we might have to deal with it.

The fear of the disease, its effects and the way it will impact on the family is only one part of it.
There is often an underlying guilt that in some way our actions may be responsible for this
having happened. Most of us will in some way or another blame ourselves, believing that we
have not been strict enough or applied enough discipline, or conversely that we have been too
strict. While these apprehensions may be quite normal the ideas aren't always rational or wellfounded.

There are usually assed to be three broad stages in any normal childhood development;
The first is observable in babies / infants. During this stage infants become focused on and
preoccupied with certain objects to the exclusion of what else is around them. If a kid's

development stalls around this point it may later show as signs of autism.

In the second recognizable stage, which is observed in older children, the child becomes
interested in a range of things at the same time and they then become incapable of
concentrating or focusing on any one thing or action for any length of time. This is the key to
ADD, as If the child stalls in their development at this stage they may later in their childhood go
on to suffer Attention Deficit Disorder (ADD).

The third stage assists a child to mature to a point from which they can comfortably focus and
voluntarily apply their attention in one certain direction for longer periods of time. They can then
alter their focus or actions as and when they have a need to. This stage is therefore a crucial
transitional stage which moulds a child for success in the classroom and in the real world.
But ADD does not only make a child or young adult incapable of focusing. It also reduces their
ability to take decisions. They can then become indecisive even in normal everyday life. An example may be that they become disoriented when crossing a road and turn back into oncoming traffic, or lose the reason why they were crossing in the first place.

At the opposite end of the scale, ADD sufferers can also become totally focused on a specific object or task. They can become consumed by it and are as a result are absolutely cut-off and

oblivious to everything else. an example of this manifesting is that they may watch the same

movie again and again without realizing, or read a certain part of a book repeatedly with no

reaction or loss of concentration. Later in life this behavior might turn into over-eating or

substance-abuse or other compulsive behavior.

Another increasingly reported variation of ADD is Attention Deficit Hyperactivity Disorder known

as ADHD. This leads to sufferers always needing to stay busy, moving from place to place or

being unable to slow down. It is increasingly being diagnosed in young teenagers. This can

drive parents mad and keep them up nights in an attempt to calm their child and entice them to

sleep. These children and young adults will find it difficult to switch off but they can experience

many of the events above. While experience of this type of patient has led Psychologists to

conclude that ADD is not a problem that a child will grow out of naturally they have also quite

strongly rejected any link with the parent causing this disorder. There is no direct causal

relationship between what a parent does an how likely a child is to develop ADD or ADHD. So if

your child is suffering from ADD stop blaming yourself, instead recognize the problem for what it

is and contact a specialist as soon as possible.

How Does ADD Impact Your Child's Education And Schooling?

There is no doubt that it is a difficult task to teach any child, but more so one suffering from
Attention Deficit Disorder. A significant number of schools have identified ADD as a legitimate
problem and have ADDressed the issue with changes in teaching methods. Substantial
developments and improvements have been made in methodology to recognize the disorder,
but there are still some which lag behind in arrangements and cannot answer an individual's
needs.

The way in which ADD can influence a classroom is often seen even before a diagnosis has
been made. It might be observed in a child reacting to his classmates, as physical reactions
such as snatching books, or in a child sitting in a corner, her mind elsewhere.
It is often a teacher who recognizes that a student is having problems attending to lessons or
are over-active. But identifying the problem is just the first step, the most difficult thing is
changing the behavior.

The treatment of ADD can only start once everyone acknowledges it. Then a diagnosis has to be made before a course of treatment is agreed. It is important early in the day to decide if medicine as a method is required, since this will determine the course of any treatment. There are some schools, which insist that a child suffering with ADD be given medicines to mitigate the effects. Some schools, however take a more patient stance and are wiling to comply with the parent's wishes.

In an ideal world, your child should be in a school which understands the effectiveness that working together as part of a team causes, by the school administration taking involvement in your child's circumstances and respecting decisions as a parent. This will assist your child in achieving the best that they can.

Regrettably some schools do not have such an open-minded vision. Communities which are smaller, and places which are poorer relative to other districts may have a habit of being too conservative. These schools can sometimes lag in catering to children who have a special need or suffer from a specific situation. ADD does make some children harder to teach. They are often more chaotic and more difficult to control. For these reasons a few schools refuse to take on and accommodate such potentially unruly children. Regardless of this you must make sure that no child is provided with a sub-standard, second-rate treatment under any circumstances.

As well as the above, some schools may run remedial classes, or classes only for students with
learning issues. Rather than these classes always assisting such children, they can be
disadvantaged by this. Children with ADD are not necessarily less intelligent at all, but classes
such as these are often of mixed abilities.

Remember though that you are the parent. You have the responsibility to achieve the best for
your child. You should always be there for him or her. If any decision taken by the school of the
class teacher goes against what you perceive to be the well-being or the best education for your
child, you should immediately discuss it with them. You may be able to come to a better plan
that will ensure the best for your child.

The Gift Of Resilience And ADD

A lack of ability to concentrate consistently Confusion makes assorted tests for various individuals. It is entirely expected for
individuals to battle while attempting to work, whether for an absence of consideration, too many intriguing interruptions or something different. At the point when you have ADD it is such a ton harder to defeat these factors, yet there is one way that is ensured to help - foster the capacity to be intense and
not set in stone.

Flexibility is characterized as 'the capacity to recuperate from or change effectively to changes or mishap.'
While relating this to grown-ups with ADD, we want to adjust the depiction marginally to be 'a capacity
to acclimate to affliction easily, to gain ground when confronted with change, to survive
hold ups, difficulties or disillusionments.'

To create as grown-ups with ADD, we should recognize the unavoidable - that we will be
confronted with issues, that we will encounter dissatisfactions and disappointments. In any case, that said we
can't permit these to stop us.

We can investigate an illustration of how flexibility applies by assessing two grown-ups with ADD, Julie and Sally.

Julie is an extremely savvy lady, however doesn't think about herself in like that. She works in a high pressure office where individuals are extremely dynamic, coming close to hyperactive. She functions as broad partner to various celebrities. One of those she works for frequently puts his missteps on her, while another supervisor over and over calls Julie unintelligent.

She spends her nights thinking about her downfalls, depleted and bothered. Accordingly she feels overpowered. While she had once been an exceptionally sure, bright lady, she has now let the remarks of a couple of individuals cut her down. While she wishes to search for a new position she questions that anybody will utilize her.

Sally is likewise a brilliant lady experiencing ADD. She struggled at school, didn't accomplish generally excellent grades, and was more than once told she was apathetic, however she continued. She moved on from secondary school and, despite the fact that her folks discouraged her from heading off to college In any case, she went. She began in junior college. At the point when she found that she could pick her own courses of study, she did pretty well.

Not set in stone to show secondary school as she needed to give a positive impact on the
individuals around her - particularly different children. Her school guide had told her that she was
silly to try and think about it. The advocate had told her that '...a individual like you can not
show secondary school. You can not handle the kids.'

Sally was frustrated for several days yet where it counts in her heart, she knew unique. She
decided not to focus on her guide and on second thought she officially mentioned an alternate
vocation's instructor whining that she ought to have an individual who might give
support. Also, she was put with one who then, at that point, reevaluated her requirements and was more steady.

Sally is presently showing secondary school history and has been for a long time. She has been designated for various honors and has been granted 'Best Secondary Teacher' two times.
Julie has lost her assurance due to what has befallen her. She has permitted the
bad introductions of others to change her viewpoints about her own value and her capacity and
she no more confidence in herself.

Sally, then again, has held her wonderful assurance.
What's more, through it all she has
had faith in herself. She doesn't let the perspectives or
confusions of others' cut her down. She
permits herself to reflect and to be Disheartened yet not
for a really long time.
Strength in grown-ups with ADD is tied in with pushing
forward. On the off chance that we might want to be
prospering developed
ups with ADD, we can't permit misfortunes to keep us
down.

How To Effectively Arrange Your Child's Therapy For ADHD

Expecting that you have proactively taken your kid or teen to a conduct trained professional and had their activities assessed by a specialist you ought to now know about the issues you face. Be that as it may, at least assuming you presently realize that you are confronted with ADHD you ought to be headed to fostering a fair treatment plan.

Properly, your youngster's clinician, specialist or doctor ought to now need to begin on a course of treatment . In any case, what is it that you want to be aware before you consent to approve and concur to a particular strategy? How do you have any idea about that what they concoct is gainful also, the most ideal choice?

The following are a couple of suggestions for you to think on. What is recorded beneath are just our thoughts, yet these have been formed subsequent to having worked with north of 1,000 kids, youthful grown-ups and youngsters with analyzed ADHD (consideration shortfall hyperactivity jumble).

1. Utilize your perspectives as a whole. Have a definite conversation with a doctor, in a perfect world your family specialist however don't be stalled by them. Any suggested strategy ought to be
all around contemplated and will contrast kid by youngster.

2. Through summer occasion we like to utilize "elective" medicines like homeopathy,
controlling eating regimen utilizing our recommended eating plans, and expanding the utilization of fundamental
unsaturated fat enhancements.

3. EEG Biofeedback preparing has likewise been found to offer incredible outcomes and ought to be seen
as an "elective" recuperating strategy for ADD. The advantage of this is that assuming these medicines are successful (and we would say they are practically 70% of the time) then, at that point, we can keep the patient away from synthetic medicines.

In the event that the underlying examination and conclusion is made later in a school year then we will generally recommend a
clinical treatment immediately for practically all patients. At the point when summer approaches we would

endeavor to diminish measurements of prescriptions and attempt the strategies above. The explanation we would utilize a
compound treatment is to attempt to 'rescue' the school year. ADHD might bring about a declining
school execution. Since prescriptions will generally work rapidly, the understudy might have the option to get through and pass classes they could somehow fall flat.

Furthermore, by evaluating the prescriptions in front of the late spring we have something to
benchmark against. We can think about the consequences of compound clinical answers for other less
intrusive medicines to be attempted and tried throughout the mid year occasions.

It merits remembering that doctors and not generally receptive while checking out
elective drugs. Specialists will generally use what they know - substance clinical arrangements -
without being willing now and again to inspect choices. Ensure that when you go to
them you are completely knowledgeable in what you need and don't allow yourself to be influenced effectively by their
obstinacy.

I did this without anyone else's help for a long time, and this is where you must come to a choice yourself on how best to assist your kid or youngster with A lack of ability to concentrate consistently Turmoil.

How Does Attention Deficit Disorder Affect Daily Life?

Living with ADD may not be simple for any youngster, teen or grown-up who has been determined to have ADD. An individual as of late determined to have ADD and foreseeing the remainder of their life may not be simple
for them. They might be uncertain the way that their illness will be impacted by age. However, over the long haul
what's more, you mature with your insight, you begin to comprehend ways of taking care of the side effects of furthermore, successfully manage ADD.

Youngsters with ADD can be neglectful, uninformed about the impacts of their activities on others and crazy, or they may effectively get diverted. They could show an excessive number of their sentiments or movement to other people. Furthermore, the side effects will remain very reliable in any event, when they go through
different ages. Anyway their capacity to deal with these side effects will work on after some time, as they get more established.

The manner in which ADD can affect on your life will to a great not set in stone by what medicine you select

to treat the issue. You could wish to counsel a specialist to give yourself a superior comprehension representing things to come impacts that taking energizers could have, and furthermore different ramifications of taking
meds.
There are numerous qualities and characteristics which are average of ADD. Individuals experiencing it ought to be ready for these. These may be troubles in their being excessively mindful of subtleties, or on the other hand issue with keeping quiet and for any time span. They may be nervous or have issues having the option to push on through and complete any given errand.

By the by it is feasible to do a scope of things to relieve the way of behaving so frequently connected with ADD. It is feasible to turn out to be more coordinated and more controlled in holding things under control. You can pick any book or a schedule to help you, however the cycle is
significant.

Schedules, timetables and arranging ought to be utilized broadly as these will show you control. As a victim of ADD you will be normally disposed to neglect, let completely go and be reckless. By utilizing a straightforward gadget, for example, a schedule you will act in a more controlled way, in a way dissimilar to your real essence. Hence you will commit less errors. You could likewise wish to turn into a piece of a gathering as this will offer Extra help. You might feel the requirement for somebody to trust in, who can comprehend you circumstance well. An individual with ADD could be an ideal sidekick since they might have the option to interface with you better than any companion or a relative, since they can uphold you just as far as possible.

Hyperactive Attention Deficit Disorder the substitute

Treatments Available

The movement away from using stimulants and medication that includes stimulants for the
treatment of ADHD has resulted in a growing market for alternative treatments. Attention Deficit
Hyperactivity Disorder has grown massively as a recognized illness in the past twenty years.
What is surprising is that there is still a limited amount of treatments available which could be
classed as 'alternative'. What follows are four powerful non-medical treatments.

1. Brainwave Bio-feedback Training

2. Behavior Modification Therapy

3. Eating / Diet Interventions

4. Nutraceutical Medicines known as Extress and Attend

These therapies can be very helpful and give significant advantages in some situations. They
are excellent when combined with the expertise of a counselor who has experience working with

ADD and ADHD. Unfortunately many counselors will have little knowledge of working with
people with these disorders.

"Attend" and "Extress" have both been found to be superb substitutes for stimulant treatment
medicines. Both of these are complicated procedures, engineered so as to achieve optimum
efficiency in brain activity in individuals experiencing problems with concentration, with
overcoming rage, with impulse control, with listening and paying attention, or with hyperactivity.
EEG Biofeedback training which is also known to many as Neuro feedback, has been around
for at least twenty years. In that sense it may be seen by some as old technology, but it has not
stood still in that time. With the development of super fast computers the technology has grown
into a recognized alternative treatment for healing of ADD. And over the time it has taken to
enhance the methods, a huge amount of study has taken place into EEG Biofeedback. There
are many websites and a wealth of information available on this including EEG Spectrum, and
other treatment alternatives are also documented well.

Eating plans and diet improvements can also have significant constructive effects on people
with ADD or with Attention Deficit Hyperactivity Disorder. Even though we are reluctant to accept that

this involvement can be applied as effectively overall as either Attend and Extress,
or a session of EEG Biofeedback methods, we certainly do consider that each person with
ADHD should try diet involvement.

A lot of people with ADD and ADHD will be assisted by nutritional supplements. Among the
most effective supplements are often Essential Fatty Acids also often known as Omega Oils. It
is also important to use supplementary minerals such as Zinc. The "Attend" nutraceutical will provide the necessary fatty acids. You also get them in Borage Oil or Flax Seed Oil. They can in
Addition be found in fish, and you can just give your child more of tuna fish to eat.

How Is Attention Deficit Disorder (ADD) Diagnosed?

While surveying regardless of whether a singular endures with A lack of ability to concentrate consistently Confusion it is a great deal harder than it might appear to laymen like ourselves. The side effects of ADD are equivalent to those of different afflictions, for example, hyperthyroidism and so on. Large numbers of the side effects are shared by all individuals eventually, so it is in many cases the size of these which analyze an individual as having ADD. So the principal significant stage in diagnosing the sickness is to counsel a restoratively prepared wellbeing supplier with respect to it.

Since what is deciphered as A lack of ability to concentrate consistently Turmoil is as yet unclear, diagnosing the disease is extremely challenging since there isn't anything which is exclusively a piece of, or absolutely beyond the extent of ADD. Albeit different associations, for example, The American Pediatrics Clinical Practice have attempted to set up rules to help individuals in perceiving the illness a great many people counting clinical experts are still frequently uncertain about such techniques.

While specialists in the past have attempted to utilize X-ray (or attractive reverberation symbolism) to dissect a
patient's mind to identify early indications of ADD, most clinical experts not longer suggest
this. Accordingly determination is in many cases presently founded fundamentally on reports of individuals near the patient, those
who see, converse with, work or live with them and have come to comprehend the patient's propensities well.

Rule distributed by the AAP (The American Foundation of Pediatrics) expects that clinical
faculty investigate a kid's way of behaving getting data from more than one area previously
they arrive at a resolution with regards to whether a kid is experiencing ADD. The specialist is hence expected to have to counsel different sources with respect to his patient's way of behaving from his school, home, the jungle gym and so forth to ensure that any determination did not depend on a youngster's conduct at one spot. This is so we can be aware for distinct that the issue is characteristic for the youngster's ordinary character and in addition to a response to what might have occurred in one spot. The rule likewise requests that a doctor use "express measures for finding" utilizing a DS-IVTR standard.

In this manner while moving toward a clinical expert for treatment, ensure that they intently

follow the headings as set by the Institute before they attempt to analyze the issue. Recollect that an issue like ADD may not be so hard to start restoring for all intents and purposes to
analyze. However, legitimate conclusion is probably going to be an initial phase in a good fix.

This is a sickness which is extremely broad in some structure, and is seen in contrasting
degrees among numerous young people. While we decide to overlook the issue and deny its
presence, It is am illness which will remain with your youngster until they are a lot more seasoned, perhaps for life. Thusly perceive the infection early and take your kid to a clinical expert for a
able conclusion and a fix.

What Does An Attention Deficit Disorder Diagnose Really Mean?

Around thirty years back, a kid was a conceived explorer, rowdy, or was said to have been
gifted with extraordinary imagination or intellectual ability, on the off chance that he was by all accounts lacking fixation, and was
restless, and imprudent. These youngsters, because of their need focus at school, were frequently
gotten out ahead, since it was believed that the work was not adequately trying to match their
abilities.

In any case, presently when a kid shows these side effects, they are for the most part determined to have ADD,
i.e., A lack of ability to concentrate consistently Confusion, and are treated at the earliest opportunity.

ADD is a seriously new disclosure, and is generally normally found among primary school young men. A average little fellow would be believed to follow up without really thinking, have an excessive amount of energy, be fretful, and
generally disapproving of packing in the class. Besides, these children generally will more often than not spend

40 or more hours seven days, before the TV, or playing computer games. It can't be rejected that numerous kids truly do have a great deal of force.

This diverted way of behaving can be made in kids due different reasons. Now and again, these variables may be very difficult, and probably won't have a say in the brain science of the kid, or the youngster's wellness conditions. For instance, the way of behaving normally saw in youngsters, experiencing ADD, might be caused because of issues of kid misuse or because of disregard. For the most part, when a youngster is determined to have ADD, a medication like Ritalin is endorsed, and the kid misuse is gone on without impedance.

The ADD side effects might connote a few extreme mental issues, for example, the bipolar jumble, profound nervousness or melancholy or even deformities in mind. Be that as it may, now and again, the causal factors perhaps very straightforward, similar to a sensitivity, aversion to the climate, lack of nourishment, or exorbitant caffeine admission.

In this way, the youngster's folks and educators, alongside their primary care physicians should regard ADD as a difficult issue, which ought to be treated with prescription as well as legitimate examination.

ADHD Treatment: Getting Started

Most guardians wonder about ADHD medicines. Is this something that your kid needs? How
might you at any point find out and at last what will the treatment include? In the event that you are one of these people, searching for a way to finding your solutions will be the main viewpoint. In
different words, treatment can come assuming you search it out yourself. The primary thing you really want to do
is to learn assuming your kid even has ADHD.

Analysis

The most vital phase in treatment for ADHD is to see whether the youngster has it. As a parent, you will need to
focus intensely on doing explore, as there is a lot of it proposed to you on the web. In any case, you
ought to likewise remember your primary care physician for your interests about your kid's way of behaving. Kids that
frequently are however to have ADHD are typically misconstrued. Assuming you observe that your kid is getting
in a tough situation more than your different kids, more than different kids in their group or more than you

believe is ordinary, then conversing with your PCP about ADHD is fundamental.

To kick the interaction off, converse with your primary care physician about your interests and afterward work to get the
replies. More often than not, youngsters should be screened by their primary care physician truly. Then, at that point,
they will converse with their social specialists, therapists and different experts that are talented in
getting to ADHD cases. The testing might be only a progression of inquiries to you and to your kid independently. Urge them to truly discuss how they feel not to attempt to reply as they naturally suspect
you need to hear. Notwithstanding these discussions, your youngster might be approached to tune in and answer
different tests.

Since every kid is very unique, the most common way of surveying their condition is probably going to be different for every youngster and each specialist. Now and again, it will be important to decide whether the kid has ADHD or on the other hand on the off chance that they maybe have a learning inability. Frequently these can be
tradable however getting the right finding implies seeking the right treatment so it ought to
take somewhat of an additional step if fundamental.

When this interaction has been finished, you will work with your primary care physician to decide the right ADHD treatment for your youngster. It could be straightforward or it very well might be perplexing. In any case, it is logical
to be definitely worth the interaction. The truth of the matter is that your kid can track down help assuming you get the interaction
begun.

ADHD Treatment: Getting Started Natural ADHD Treatment

For those that are experiencing ADHD, there are numerous treatment choices out there. Some individuals could do without to utilize synthetic prescriptions to treat conditions like this. These people will endeavor to search out the assist that they with requiring in treating ADHD with elective cures. There are a few superb home grown cures that can assist with advancing wellbeing and well being to those that are searching for some different option from prescriptions. Despite the fact that you ought to never quit taking any sort of drug endorsed to you by a specialist, you might discover some help in these natural cures too.

One method for knowing whether a home grown item has demonstrated to be any sort of help depending on the prerequisite that you are confronted with is to see research studies. In certain examinations that have been finished around the world over the most recent quite a long while, there are a few Chinese natural cures that have displayed to give kids worked on prosperity and even treat ADD and ADHD really. One natural cure that does this incorporates home grown parts including Chinese throwax root, skullcap root, ginseng root, red jujube leafy foods fixings. The mix of the fixings was said to give a quieting impact on the kid.

One more equation that is utilized for ADHD treatment offers an enemy of burdensome recipe and treatment. Here, you will find fixings like St. John's Wort, Kava, Chamomile, Lavender natural oils, Skullcap, Signseng, and orange medicinal oil. This blend is said to accommodate a treatment for ADHD too.

Ginkgo is one spice that you might track down in a portion of these natural cures. This sort of spice is said to further develop the blood stream to the mind. By expanding the vascular flow there, it is said to give further developed memory as well as further developing fixation.

Hawthorne is another treatment choices. Here, the objective is to fortify the heart and the circulatory framework. It is utilized in numerous old Chinese meds to quiet the brain. Furthermore, spices like skullcap, lemon demulcent and oats are utilized to assist with giving a nerve tonic that will assist with sustaining as well as proposition ordinariness to the sensory system, working on the singular's general serenity and clearness. Natural cures have been utilized for a long time to treat conditions like ADHD. Attempting to consolidate a portion of these cures can frequently be useful. As they are regular, they are probably not going to make aftereffects the person as well for however long they are taken as they are coordinated.

Medications for ADHD: A Summary

Finding the right ADHD treatment implies tracking down the right mix of treatment choices for you. Every youngster or grown-up that has ADHD will get himself a piece extraordinary in his circumstance. Very much like some other condition, equipping the treatment of that condition to its particulars is fundamental.

However, there is a generally huge closeness between the medicines advertised. That will be just each finding and treatment will accompany medicine help, conduct help along with instructive mediations.

Prescriptions

The principal thing that comes to person's psyches when they here prescription is ailment. The truth of the matter is that youngsters and grown-ups that experience the ill effects of ADHD will encounter conditions that dislike others. They frequently see things or learn things in a remarkable manner. Intermittently this expectation to learn and adapt is something that should be surely known before meds can be regulated. There are

numerous prescriptions that are accessible to support assisting the singular arrangement with the circumstances that
their ADHD is causing. Some are very mind, some are areas of strength for extremely. Some deal not very many
secondary effects, others many. Your PCP will work with you to decide the right prescription for
your necessities.

Conduct Treatment

Showing the kid how to adapt to different circumstances with regards to their ADHD can be
enormously valuable. Youngsters that comprehend how to respond when they are baffled, furious or
misconstrued can figure out how to all the more likely control their way of behaving and afterward make more progress in their
treatment. However, conduct treatment is frequently insufficient all alone. Adding drug to the
interaction can offer more rewards.

Instructive Intercession

Training is likewise vital. Assuming the person with ADHD comprehends what ADHD is and
understands the advantages of his condition, he can all the more likely make progress. Those that don't have the foggiest idea

what's going on have minimal possibility having worked on confidence and may try and battle
conduct and drug medicines that are hoping to work on his condition. A blend of these treatment strategies is generally the best strategy for the
individual that has ADHD. Albeit many guardians battle the possibility of drugs, it is frequently a
fundamental piece of permitting the youngster to make progress with his condition. Regardless of who the individual is, assist with canning be found for ADHD in the method of medicines when all parts of the circumstance are thought about.

Therapies for ADHD: Medications

ADHD medicines frequently incorporate some type of treatment drug. There are a few
prescriptions available that are utilized broadly to assist youngsters as well as grown-ups who with having
been determined to have treatment. A considerable lot of these treatment choices are dependent upon the person's
response to them. In some cases this implies that you should attempt a few preceding seeing as the right decision for your condition. Finding the right medicine implies that ADHD can be to a lesser degree a
issue for the individual and they can work on their everyday capabilities, particularly at school
or on the other hand work.

Most drugs for ADHD are energizers. Numerous people don't grasp this as numerous
that experience the ill effects of ADHD are very twisted up and worked up. However, dissimilar to those that would take a
energizer to give them more energy, the energizers work another way for the individual with
ADHD. They work by invigorating the mind in a particular region to assist them with acquiring advantages such

as better abilities to focus, more control rather than drive choices and more clarity of mind in the undertakings
they need to achieve. These prescriptions work by assisting the cerebrum with having more prominent self guideline.

Here are the absolute most normal meds for ADHD medicines.
Methylphenidate: These are tracked down in Ritalin, Metadate, Methylin and Focalin. These are
typically required three times each day after feasts. There are others including Ritalin LA and Focalin
XR that are long portions that will reach out as long as 12 hours.

Amphetamines: Here, you might find decisions, for example, Dexedrine that is taken a few times for every day, ADDerall which is both accessible in short and longer periods and others.
Different drugs for ADHD treatment including Atomoxetine, Bupropion which is all the more well known as Wellbutrin, Benzphetamine which is significantly less strong, Provigil which is a new decision, and Clonidine.

There is a ton of experimentation that goes into the assurance of the right drug for an
person that experiences ADHD. The best instrument that can be given to them is exact

analysis as well as determination at taking the prescriptions. When something isn't right with the prescription, they ought to tell their PCP at that moment so an option can be found. ADHD medicines with prescription ought to likewise be assisted with conduct and instructive help too. The blend can permit youngsters and grown-ups to track down additional responses to their questions and generally speaking improved results to their requirements.

What Takes Place Throughout ADHD Treatments When Medication Is Insufficient?

Commonly, people with ADHD don't answer all around ok with the meds to offer
them enough control and direction over their circumstance. At the point when this is the situation, everybody
involved can end up being very disappointed and stressed. However, there is little uncertainty that having the right
devices and the right schooling about the condition can assist you with getting the achievement you want in tracking down the right ADHD treatment.

Some of the time, prescription isn't the main response accessible. While any youngster metal grown-up that is taking
prescription for ADHD ought to take constantly it except if they converse with their primary care physician first, it very well may be
very advantageous to ADD different sorts of medicines to the crease too. It is normal for there to be

contrasts in patient to patient, your most memorable undertaking in assisting somebody with getting past ADHD
issues is to track down an effective and experienced specialist. All to frequently the family specialist is the one
passed on to settle on the conclusions about ADHD with the kid. Finding somebody that practices would be able go with the medicine and the conduct decisions better for them.

Furthermore, when meds don't appear to be sufficient treatment for ADHD, it is moreover
critical to consider feelings of anxiety, profound injury (a few kids with ADHD are discouraged
or on the other hand any other way confronting nervousness that can deteriorate the side effects) as well as diet. These things
can set off expanded ADHD side effects that can cause the prescriptions to appear as though they are not
Adequately working. However, these circumstances can be treated too.

Substitute Medicines

There are a few elective medicines to ADHD prescriptions. Those that don't need their
kid to take drug or don't feel that they need to take them themselves can utilize these
elective choices to offer some assistance. A few examinations have found that those that don't eat a

adjusted diet that is plentiful in minerals and nutrients are bound to encounter ADHD. In
Expansion, there are those medicines which are not demonstrated yet can be useful. That's what some case drinking gentle energizer items like Caffeine filled beverages can give a portion of the quieting impacts of ADHD meds. There are home grown supplements that are accessible that too support help for ADHD.It is valid that occasionally drug don't function admirably enough for the person. That doesn't actually

mean, however that there isn't any treatment or help for them. Working with a specialist that is talented in the field can offer more outcome in tracking down the right answer for the youngster. There are numerous hypotheses and false impressions out there. However, with the talented specialist, you can see as the treatment choices that are ideal for you.

Therapies for ADHD: The Diet

When considering the right ADHD treatment for a child or an adult, it can be important to take a
look at their specific diet. Those that find that medication do not work, do not want to take
medication or are looking for Added benefits with the medications should take a look at the diet
of the individual that has ADHD. Studies have shown that many individuals that have ADHD
also have diet deficiency. Other studies have shown that some individual's that do have ADHD
have a body chemistry that reacts to some food products in the wrong way, leading to worsened
symptoms.

It is essential to take a good look at the diet of the individual and adjust it if at all possible. Diet
modification can help to improve the ADHD that an individual has, improving their life quality
and lessening symptoms. One of the most well known types of diets to consider is that of the
Feingold Diet. In this diet, the idea is to pull out some of the most unnatural of elements that are
commonly found in food today. This may including such things as salicylates, food colorings
and flavors that are not naturally there, as well as preservatives that are not natural.

Modifying the diet can be quite troublesome to individuals that face ADHD. Many times,
children are the hardest hit by this change. Removing foods that are packed with preservatives,
artificial flavorings and other poor quality ingredients can be difficult as it is in many of the
children's favorite foods. The more that they consume of these products though, the more
troublesome their health and their ADHD can be.

One effective method to getting past this problem is to keep the diet in mind as a food change
for the entire family. As none of these ingredients has shown to be good for the body, everyone
can benefit by not consuming things like junk food chips, cookies, and other candies. Limiting
them can also be helpful. Working to incorporate better health benefiting products is also a
good thing.

There are some studies that show that improving the diet of a child with more whole foods,
including foods that are not processed or refined can help to improve their ADHD symptoms.
Although it is not thought of as causing the ADHD in the first place, there is evidence that an
improved diet can lead to improvements overall for the child or adult that suffers from ADHD.

The Negative Effects Of ADHD Therapies

When a youngster is determined to have ADHD, treatment choices will introduce themselves. Since there are an ever increasing number of youngsters being determined every day to have this condition, there is little uncertainty
that there will be a few times when some unacceptable treatment is introduced to the kid. It is
fundamental that guardians take a lot of watchfulness in managing these issues. The most ideal way to
do that is to safeguard that you are completely instructed with regards to ADHD as well as the prescriptions that are given to the person. With schooling about the terrible side of ADHD
medicines, the right treatment can be helpful without Added issues.

Incidental effects.

One thing that should be considered is the way that there are incidental effects to a significant number of the drugs that are utilized to treat ADHD. Most medications will make a few side impacts, yet some are
much more awful than others. While your PCP will let you know the particular incidental effects for your specific medicine, there are some that are more normal in these prescriptions. For

model, a few youngsters have a deficiency of craving while the meds are in their frameworks.

Different side effects that can be normal incorporate sleep deprivation, anxiety, weight reduction, issues with falling off the drugs and emotional episodes. ADHD prescription secondary effects offer a wide scope of advantages and frequently these advantages can offset the symptoms of the medication.

Finding support

At the point when you feel that the symptoms of a treatment are irksome converse with your PCP. He or she might suggest that the measurement of the meds be expanded or brought down. Some meds influence a few youngsters unique. There are a few unique kinds of meds that however, can be utilized to treat ADHD. So on the off chance that one prescription isn't functioning admirably or the incidental effects are problematic, your primary care physician ought to be reached as there are different arrangements.

Guardians of youngsters that are recently determined to have ADHD ought to give close consideration to the prescriptions that the youngster takes. At times it can require a few days for the prescription to enter the circulation system enough to see a distinction. Here and there insufficient drug is endorsed.

Likewise, guardians ought to monitor any exceptional changes or whatever is irksome or

troubling in their youngster. With this data they can work intimately with their youngster's primary care physicians to
track down the best portion of medicine. Remember your youngster's instructors for this interaction also.

Milton Keynes UK
Ingram Content Group UK Ltd.
UKHW012133010224
437116UK00011B/753